YOGA FOR THE DESK JOCKEY

This book makes an ideal gift for employees, associates, suppliers, and clients

as a sales promotion reward, loyalty reward, fundraising vehicle, and educational tool.

Special editions catered to your organization can be created to meet your specific needs.

For more information please contact us at 403.229.2617 or through our website at

www.yogaforthedeskjockey.com

Other books and e-books by Susi Hately Aldous

ANATOMY AND ASANA: THE SACROILIAC JOINTS

ANATOMY AND ASANA: THE KNEES

ANATOMY AND ASANA: PREVENTING YOGA INJURIES

ANATOMY AND ASANA: SHOULDER ISSUES BOOK 1

www.anatomyandasana.com

5% of revenues are given to charities supporting health and wellbeing.

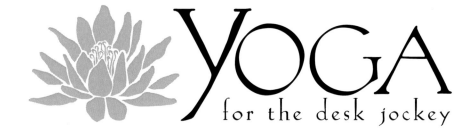

YOGA
for the desk jockey

by

Susi Hately Aldous

PUBLISHED BY SHA-PRESS
www.sha-press.com
To reach the author directly, please visit www.yogaforthedeskjockey.com.
Editor: Patricia MacDonald
Book design by Janine Mackinnon Art & Design
Printed in Canada by Blitzprint

DISCLAIMER
The purpose of this book is to provide
information for desk workers on the subject of yoga.
This book does not offer any medical advice to the reader and is
not intended as a replacement for appropriate health care and treatment.
For such advice, readers should consult their health care practitioners.

TO DAVE AND SADIE

CARA

AND ALL MY CLIENTS

THANK YOU

HOW TO USE THIS BOOK

 have written this book with the intention of enabling you to experience less pain, less irritation, more inspiration, and more calmness while at work.

To inspire this, I have designed and laid out the material according to a standard workday. There are strategies you can use upon waking and on the way to work, techniques for your breaks, and ideas for lunch. There are suggestions for your drive home and ways to release work-related tension while at home. We cover yoga poses, breathing, and meditation techniques designed for your body, mind, and soul, creating a unified whole for you.

PLEASE TAKE CARE OF YOURSELF

The following practices and strategies have been taught to thousands of desk workers over the past 7 years with very successful results. As you practice, please keep in mind that your body changes from day to day, and you alone know your body best. What you do one day may not work on another. Please move with awareness, with breath, and in your pain-free range of motion. To help you do this, please read the tips on moving, breathing, and relaxing on the next page.

Have a great day at work!

Susi

TIPS ON RELAXING, MOVING, & BREATHING WHILE AT WORK

1. Before you begin any of these moves, take a moment and settle. Feel yourself breathing, and continue to easily and gently breathe while you are moving into, staying in, or moving out of the pose or technique.
2. Do the techniques that serve you. If something doesn't resonate with you, do what does resonate.
3. Be sure to move in your pain-free range of motion. This can sometimes be difficult to distinguish, so to help, try this – if you are holding your breath, clenching your jaw, scrunching up your face, or holding extra tension while you are moving, then you are moving too far and/or too fast. Please ease out and find your breath and sense of relaxation once again.
4. The more you can easily breathe your soft, natural, normal breath, the more your body will relax. And in the context of these exercises and techniques, the more you relax, the stronger you will become.
5. Please don't force yourself. Forcing will only make you weaker.
6. If you have questions, I'd love to hear from you. Please email me through www.yogaforthedeskjockey.com.

The great mind knows the power of gentleness. – Robert Browning

CONTENTS

CONTENTS continued on next page

CONTENTS

The Practices

These practices are simple

strategies and techniques that you

can use to release tension,

gain strength, and

improve flexibility

so that you

can experience less pain,

less strain, and more comfort

while at work.

GOOD MORNING!

nitiating a breathing or gentle yoga program in the morning can be the most time-efficient and luxurious way to integrate yoga into your day. When you do simple yoga moves in the morning, your daily energy will improve.

How to do it:

1. Begin on your back, knees bent or straight, hands on your belly. Take five easy breaths through your nose, and feel how your breath is moving through your torso in the following places:
   - Just below your navel
   - At the base of your breastbone
   - At the notch of your collar bones
2. Notice if your breath is full and easy, if it is narrow or thin, empty, shallow, deep, or slim. Be okay with whatever the experience is.
3. Next take one knee gently to your belly, keeping your shoulders and neck relaxed. Imagine that you can breathe into your hip.
4. Breathe five breaths, then switch sides and repeat. When you are complete, rest back and check your breathing. When ready, roll over and carry on with your day.

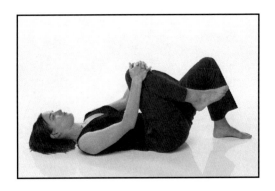

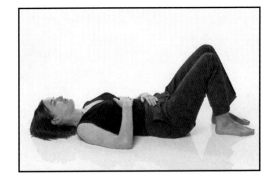

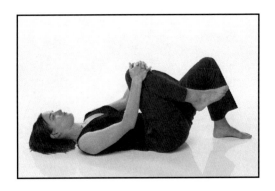

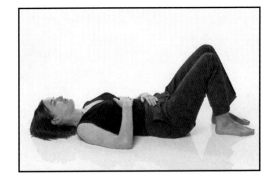

Flow fact:

Breathing, relaxing,

and releasing can

bring more vitality to

your day than even

the most steaming

cup of coffee.

THE MORNING PROGRAM

orning programs are a way to settle in, to take note of yourself, to feel the inner tune that is driving you on any given day.

How to do it:

1. Choose a place that you love. It does not have to be in your house. Some of the best morning sessions occur in the park during a walk or by the water.

2. Become aware of your breath and the sensations in your body. Be sure you are not judging how good – or not good – this feels. This is a time to notice, not a time to create a reason for it or to make an excuse. Just notice the myriad sensations moving through your body.

3. Move at a pace your body likes. Be aware if your mind is wanting to "kick your ass" into shape. If your body is tired and worn out, lying over a bolster or taking your legs up the wall can be the most rejuvenating experience. Distinguish the difference between your body's desires and your mind's desires. Follow your body.

4. Notice the inner knowing that bubbles up. If you stick with your breath, your sense of inner knowing will become stronger. Follow those "hits" and see what happens. Most likely, you'll be pleasantly surprised.

The first hour of the morning is the rudder of the day.

– Henry Ward Beecher, American congressional clergyman, religious writer, and reformer

When I was completing my first book, *Anatomy and Asana: Preventing Yoga Injuries,* there was a hectic time of final editing, design, and printing. I knew this was not the time to become sick or run down. So I became extra conscious in how I planned my day – beginning with my "morning program."

My morning program was my chance to check in – to notice my breath, to notice my body, and to be aware of how both were feeling. Some mornings, my body expressed anxiety and doubt with its inner vibrations; other mornings, when uncertainty came knocking, my breath held static, solid, and unmoving in my chest; on yet other mornings, when the book process was in a noticeably forward-moving direction, I could feel my breath flowing freely, my body easily releasing tension as I stretched from one yoga pose into another.

In all, my morning program helped me tune into my awareness and to own my state of mind and body so that my various fears and doubts weren't affecting others in my home or in the studio. The tribulations became humorous anecdotes, and the successes definite celebrations. Without question, my morning program was a key to completing my first book.

Flow fact:

Taking time to be aware of the sensations in your body – and then following them –

will strengthen your intuition and your clarity and will lead you to success faster than

if you ignore the sensations and act only according to your mental chatter.

ON THE WAY TO WORK

 ou can build up a reservoir of energy as you drive, ride, or walk to work, or even while standing on the bus. As you practice, you will feel your inner core becoming stronger and your posture more upright, plus a gentle bounce to your step.

How to do it:

1. While you are sitting or standing, gently contract your urinary muscles. Release. Repeat – contract, release, contract, release.
2. Be sure your anal muscles are relaxed and uninvolved.
3. Once you are comfortable doing this, try to statically hold the contraction for one or two breaths. Progressively increase the length of time you contract these muscles while still being able to breathe easily through your nose. The key is being able to breathe easily.
4. You want to make sure you are not holding excessive tension in your body (namely your chest or jaw) while you are doing this exercise.

Flow fact:

Building inner stability is a key factor in helping tight shoulders release,

sore necks find ease, and achy lower backs find relief.

GETTING PRESENT: PREPARING FOR A DAY AT WORK

A simple four-step process completed at the beginning of your workday can help prevent pain and tension from creeping into your body later in the day.

How to do it:

1. As you sit in front of your computer, feel your butt planted on the chair or ball, your feet planted on the floor or footrest.
2. Maintain your upright posture and go inside for a moment. Without changing your physical integrity, let the inside of your body relax. Relax your anal muscles.
3. Become aware of the moment – your body, your breath through your nose, the actions and energy of others around you.
4. Maintaining this level of awareness, pause. Wait for your own innate wisdom to flow through you.

What do you feel, see, or hear?

Business people need to slow down and be more reflective.

— Tom Durel, management consultant

Taking a Break:
Release Your Shoulders

After just a few hours in front of a computer, I always find it amazing to notice how the tightness quietly creeps up – into the shoulders, the upper back, the neck, the jaw. While the mind is creatively spinning out new ideas or answers to questions, in creeps the physical discomfort, so stealthily, just outside of conscious awareness . . . until a few hours later there is a need to move, to release tight muscles, or to get a glass of water.

The following shoulder releases are in honour of the discomfort that surreptitiously *crrreeeeps* in. Just as easily as it moves in, we're going to move it out.

Which exercises should I do?
Try them all at first. Continue with the ones that allow you to breathe through your nose and that make your body feel really good as you do them.

If you don't stretch, you don't know where your edge is.

– Sara Little Turnbull,

Stanford graduate school of business,

director of the process of

change laboratory

ARM CIRCLES OVERHEAD

This exercise feels so good, and it offers the added benefit of some arm strengthening. Be sure to breathe while you perform the motions.

How to do it:

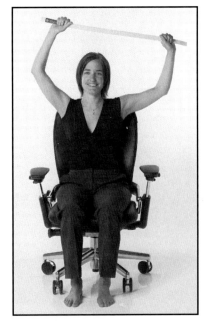

1. Take a strap in your hands so that the hands are more than shoulder-width apart.
2. Raise your hands above your head, keeping your elbows bent. Begin to circle your arms.
3. Relax your jaw and breathe through your nose.
4. If the movement feels good, and you are breathing easily, gently straighten your arms.
5. Find the ease, circle a few more times, then switch sides.

CHEST RELEASE

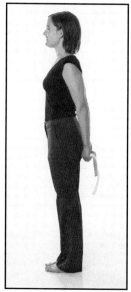

This move will help release the chest muscles that get tight after a few hours in a slouched posture.

How to do it:

1. Standing near the edge of your chair, put your hands behind you and grasp a strap. Relaxing your jaw and breathing easily, *gently* slide the lower tips of your shoulder blades toward each other and down your back. Breathe through your nose five times.
2. Release. You may feel this in your chest or slightly down your arms. If there is tingling or numb-like sensations, ease out immediately.

You must learn to be still in the midst of activity, and to be vibrantly alive in repose. – Indira Gandhi

SHOULDER ROLLS

The shoulder blades can become stuck when we sit for long periods of time. Shoulder rolls help release them.

How to do it:

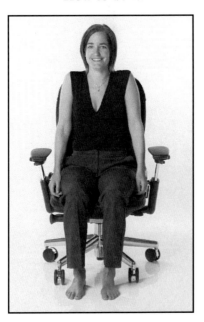

1. Sit with your weight equally on your sitting bones.
2. Inhale, raising your shoulders and shoulder blades to your ears.
3. Exhale, sliding your shoulder blades toward each other and down your back. Keep your arms quiet, moving mostly at your shoulder blades. Repeat about 5 to 10 times, as long as you are relaxed and you are breathing easily through your nose.
4. If there is any pain – like "knife searing" – ease out of the movement.

ELBOW CIRCLES

lbow circles help release most of the muscles connecting to the shoulder. As you do them, you will also feel your breath release.

How to do it:

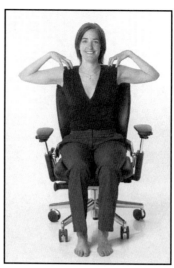

1. In sitting or standing, touch your fingers to your shoulders.
2. Make circles with your elbows; inhale as you initiate the circle in a backward direction, and begin your exhale about halfway through the motion as you move your elbows to complete the circle.
3. If you are standing/sitting perpendicular to a wall, imagine you can draw circles on the wall with your elbows.
4. Keep the shoulders as quiet as possible.
5. If you experience elbow pain as you move, make the circles smaller, be sure you are breathing, and check to see that your shoulders are quiet and not too rigid.

EAGLE POSE

 your arms are your wings. Imagine you are perched on a branch, with your wings close to your body. This move will help release between the neck and shoulders; and between the shoulders, arms and upper back.

How to do it:

1. In sitting, place your hands out in front of you, palms up.
2. Cross your arms at the elbows so that the elbows are on top of each other. **If your arms are unable to nestle one on top of the other, hold one elbow with the opposite hand. You just need some time for your shoulders to release.
3. Move your hands, turning your thumbs toward your face. Relax your shoulders; relax your jaw.
4. Breathe five calm and easy breaths through your nose.

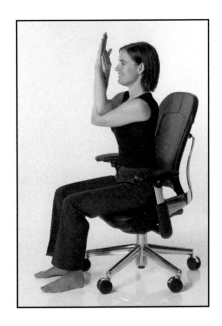

SHOULDER RELEASE WITH STRAP

his position is doubly good in that it releases the back of the arm on one side and the front of the arm/shoulder and chest on the other.

How to do it:

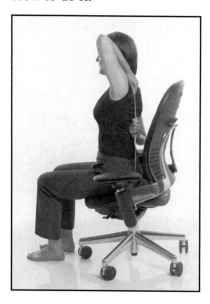

1. In sitting, place a strap over your left shoulder.
2. Raise your left arm beside your ear. Bend it at the elbow, and gently grab your strap.
3. Move your right arm behind your body, and gently grab your strap. **If you can't grab your strap, please don't strain. Just rest your hand on your back in a comfortable position.
4. Imagine your collar bones are broadening.
5. Breathe through your nose twice (you can work up to 10 easy breaths).
6. Release and switch to the opposite side.

SHOULDER AND BACK RELEASE USING CHAIR

his position will help release your shoulders along with the hips, back of the legs, and your back. An all in one.

How to do it:

1. Lean forward from your hips and grasp the top of the chair. **If you are prone to back pain, either bend your knees or use the wall, or a shelf, so that you don't lean forward as much.

2. Breathe through your nose. Let yourself settle into the pose.

3. Keeping the rest of your body still, bend your left elbow toward the floor. Imagine that the space between your shoulder blades is getting bigger and the lower tip of your left shoulder blade is moving down and outward. Release. Do the same with the right. Move one elbow at a time, keeping your torso still.

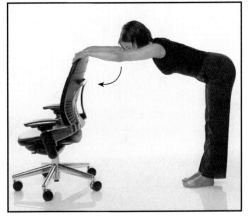

4. Repeat two to five times each side, then return to standing.

THE TWO-ARM SHAKE

 This two-arm shake will lead you toward liberating your shoulders.

How to do it:

1. Every hour or so, while seated, let your arms drop to your sides.
2. Shake your fingers and wrists, add the elbows, and finally add the shoulders. Continue for 15 seconds, and work up to 1 minute. Relax your jaw.
3. Find yourself having a hard time getting the elbows and shoulders involved? Stay with it; they just need to loosen up.

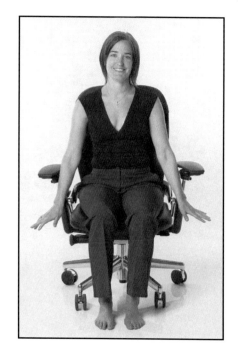

UPPER SHOULDER/NECK RELEASE

This move can help release tight muscles related to tension headaches and eye strain.

How to do it:

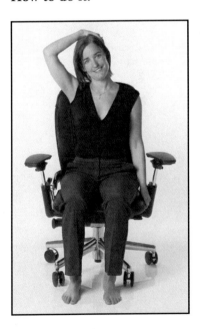

1. While seated, gently grasp the side of the seat cushion of the office chair with your left hand in order to anchor the shoulder girdle.
2. As you breathe in, place your right hand on top of your head, slightly toward the left ear.
3. While slowly breathing out, *gently* bring the right ear toward the right shoulder. Stay for two to five breaths.
4. Switch to the other side and repeat.

YOGA FOR LUNCH

 n a culture focused on the "what" of eating, we can sometimes forget about the "how" of eating.

How to do it:

1. Slow down, sit down, and settle. If you have to be at your desk, clear away the files and papers. Turn your computer monitor off. Close your books. Put away the newspaper. Let this moment nourish you.
2. Breathe. Look at your food. Be aware of what you are about to eat.
3. As you chew, notice. Notice the flavour, the texture, the temperature. Indulge in the pleasure; in the solace of eating enough; and in the calm, light, and vital sense of energy that comes from the feeling of not being over-full.

Whether you eat your meal in 5 minutes, 15 minutes, or an hour, transition yourself back to work – take a moment, a breath, or a walk. Moving back into work with ease and breath allows your digestive system to absorb and eliminate what it needs to, which in turn will give you ultimate energy and well-being.

The most important blessing I can
think of before eating is the
simple act of being present.
It's so easy to rush to the table
and devour your food while being
everything but there.
Who wants to eat your errands,
your income taxes, or your emails?
By centering on the breath for
even two or three cycles
I come back home to myself,
and can bring my attention
more fully to the gift of taste,
nourishment and abundance
which is so easy to take for granted.

— Joan Borysenko, former Harvard medical scientist and psychologist

Taking a Break: Release Your Hips

As you are reading this, uncross your legs and relax your forehead. Feel yourself breathing. The following yoga moves will help release your hips and ease the tension from your spine and lower back, as well as strengthen your legs.

Which exercises should I do?
On first read, try them all; then do the ones that enable you to breathe easily through your nose and allow you to relax.

Flow fact: *You will become stronger if you release your tight hips.*

SITTING HIP RELEASE

People often say "ohhh" and smile when they do this one. Releasing the hips and back never felt so good.

How to do it:

Be sure that when you move into position, you move from your hips, not your spine. If you experience inner knee sensations, immediately come out of the pose.

1. Begin in sitting, both feet on the floor.
2. Raise your right knee toward you and hold it with your hands. This may be a good stretch for you. If so, stay here and breathe. If your body wants more, be sure you are breathing easily and continue.
3. Take the right ankle and place it on the left knee. If there is right knee pain, continue to hold your right knee in a position where there is no pain. If your knee is okay, release your grip.
4. As you exhale, think of keeping your collar bones broad and your breastbone lifted gently, and lean forward from your hips.
5. Stay in the position for between 2 and 10 easy, calm breaths.
6. As you inhale, return to start.
7. Repeat twice, then switch sides.

SITTING HAMSTRING RELEASE

This move will help your hamstrings (back of thighs) and your calves.

How to do it:

When you move into the position, move from your hips, not your spine.

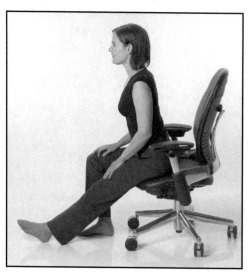

1. Sitting at the edge of your chair, straighten your left leg in front of you. Inhale.
2. As you exhale, move forward from your hips, keeping your collar bones broad and your breastbone lifted gently. Relax your head.
3. Stay in the position for between 2 and 10 breaths.
4. If your body wants more, gently and slowly turn your toes to the ceiling.
5. Inhale and return to sitting. Repeat twice, then switch sides.

ONE-LEG HIP RELEASE

his exercise combines balance, strength, and release. A good one if you are feeling anxious.

How to do it:

Come into standing and hold the wall, the back of your chair, or your desk for support.

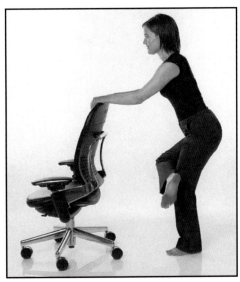

1. In standing, lift your right ankle onto your left knee.
2. Gently bend your left knee. Breathe through your nose.
3. Relax your jaw and your shoulders, and breathe easily for 5 to 10 breaths.
4. You may feel some leg strengthening as well as hip releasing.
5. Be sure there is no knee or back pain. If there is, ease up out of the position to a place where you feel no pain.
6. Switch sides.

STANDING SIDE BEND

If your day began at 9:00 a.m., this one is terrific at about 2:00 p.m. when you are feeling cramped from sitting for 5 hours.

How to do it:

1. Stand equally on both feet.
2. Inhale and raise your left hand to your left ear. Let your right arm rest along your right leg.
3. Exhaling, lean to your right, doing your best to keep the weight through your feet equal on the floor.
4. If you want more, straighten your left arm alongside your head.
5. Be sure you don't feel this in your back. If you do, ease up a little.
6. On your inhale, return to start. Repeat on other side.

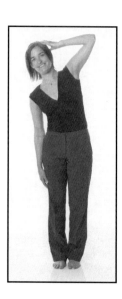

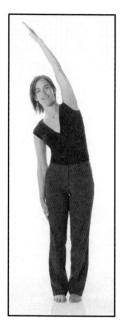

Notice that the stiffest
tree is most easily cracked,
while the bamboo or willow
survives by bending
with the wind.

– Bruce Lee

STRENGTHENING YOUR LEGS AND BUTT

When we sit, the muscles of our thighs, butt, and arms become weaker. This pose, called Chair Pose, adds some strength to these key areas.

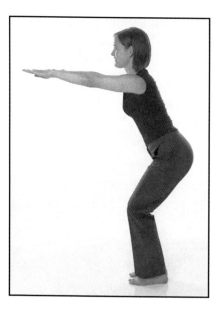

How to do it:

1. Come into standing, with your weight equally over both feet. Relax your toes.
2. Inhale, raising your arms to shoulder height.
3. Exhale, bending your knees over your ankles. Stay for two breaths.
4. On your third inhale, return to standing. Repeat two more times, as long as your breath is easy and your jaw relaxed. Be sure there is no knee pain. If there is, ease up slightly to a position where your knees are pain free.

STANDING HIP RELEASE

If you cross your legs when you sit, this pose is terrific for stretching tight inner thighs.

How to do it:

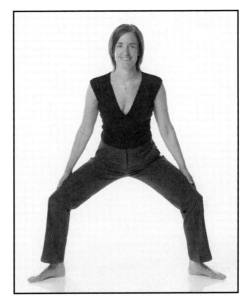

1. Point your left foot to "11:00" and your right foot to "1:00."

2. Exhale, bending your knees over your ankles, being sure there is no knee pain. Place your hands on the outside of your thighs. Press the thighs into your hands (notice that your knees move on top of your ankles when you do this). Relax your jaw.

3. Relax your shoulders, and breathe three to five breaths through your nose.

BRINGING CLOSURE:
FINISHING YOUR DAY AT WORK

The 5 minutes you spend consciously finishing your day can be the most effective time management, stress management, and day-planning activity you can do for yourself. Acting as a transition from your day at work to your evening at home, it gives you a chance to take note of what was completed, what wasn't completed, and overall how the day went.

How to do it:

1. Clear your desk.
2. Sit or stand and breathe. Feel your breath in your body. How does it feel?
3. Ask yourself, how did your day go – how did it feel?
4. Take note of what you wanted to accomplish. Did you accomplish what you wanted to?
5. Next, note what you need to do tomorrow. Include the items not already completed. Write them down on a piece of paper. Choose the three most important tasks, and asterisk them. Use those to focus your day tomorrow.
6. Place the piece of paper on your desk, your chair, or your keyboard so that you will see it tomorrow.

HEADING HOME

 eading home by car, train, bus, or foot provides a great opportunity to check in with yourself to assess interaction between your day at work and your body, mind, and soul.

How to do it:

Be mindful of what is happening in your body and mind. Also known as mindfulness, this technique enables you to see/hear/feel the mental chatter in your mind and sensations in your body that can be clouded when fatigued. All you do is observe. It is as if you are clearing away the cloud and penetrating into what is really going on "now." But you must do it without judgment, without trying to figure out anything. Just notice. As you do, something amazing happens. Time slows down, and a sense of clarity and calmness emerges.

Nothing is more practical than for people to deepen themselves.

— Peter Koestenbaum, philosopher

AN EVENING MEDITATION

editation is an amazing stress buster, mostly because it gets you out of your mental chatter and into the stillness within.

How to do it:

Take 3 to 5 minutes to start.

1. Begin sitting, standing, or walking. Feel yourself breathing. Feel yourself inhaling and exhaling. Just watch the breath come into your body and leave your body. Try focusing on your nostrils and feeling the air come in and go out.
2. As you notice yourself being pulled away from your breath, gently pull yourself back to the sensations in your body – to your nostrils, your breath. Continue to practice.
3. When you are complete, take a few normal breaths, thank yourself, and carry on with your day. If you are doing this every day, notice what happens over the course of a week, and then let me know. I welcome your comments about your journey into meditation (email through www.yogaforthedeskjockey.com).

Flow fact: As you develop your facility with meditation, your immune system will become stronger, anxiety will drop, and sleep and digestion will improve.

Is Your Mind Chatter Getting the Best of You?

Remember, mind chatter is just that. Mind chatter. It has nothing to do with you, it is just the thoughts and distractions that move about in our minds. The training of meditation allows you to notice when you get pulled away by your thoughts and then bring yourself back to what is real – your breath, the sensations in your body. That's it. Know that you will wander with your thoughts. This is just what happens.

The only difference between a novice and experienced meditator is the experienced meditator can bring herself back to her point of focus faster than a novice meditator.

The reverse side

also has a reverse side.

— Japanese proverb

Ergonomics

Relaxing, moving, and breathing while at work

are important components for a healthier, happier,

and less tense you. But in order to really be comfortable,

you need to perform the techniques that work

for you *and* know how to set up your workstation,

how to sit, and how to assess your posture.

Here are three principles to follow to help you

further enhance your comfort.

SETTING UP YOUR WORKSTATION

Whether you are 4 feet or 6 feet tall, long legged and short bodied, short legged and long bodied, there are ways to set up your workstation to suit your body type and reduce physical strain and discomfort. Follow these ideas and combine them with the movements and breathing techniques that work for you, and you will be on your way to being pain free.

How to do it:

1. Set your chair so that your feet are on the floor or on your footrest and your knees, hips, and elbows are at about 90 degrees. Sit on the whole chair, and let your chair back support you.
2. Ensure there is a fist width between the front edge of the seat and your knees.
3. Allow your fingers to comfortably rest on your keyboard with your wrists in neutral. Be sure your keyboard is directly in front of you. Let your wrists be supported by the wrist support.
4. Place your mouse next to your keyboard.
5. Set your monitor about an arm's length away and directly in front of you. Position the screen so that your chin is not excessively pointing up or down.
6. Relax your shoulders; relax your jaw. Let your spine lift effortlessly to the ceiling.
7. Breathe.

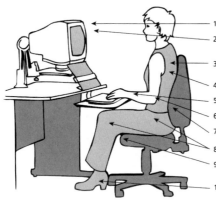

1. Top of monitor parallel to the desk surface (i.e. flat)

2. Top of screen parallel to eye level (to maintain neutral neck posture – monitor may be lower if wearing bifocal or progressive lenses)

3. Back and shoulder blades supported against the backrest of chair, backrest locked

4. Relax the shoulders and breathe

5. Wrists straight, keyboard and mouse on same surface

6. Elbows bent at 90 degrees, by side of body

7. Lumbar support at correct height ("in small of back")

8. 90 degree angle in hips an knees

9. Three-finger gap between the knee and the front edge of the chair's seat pan

10. Feet flat on the floor (or a footrest)

Copyright Anderson Ergonomics Consulting Inc. 2004

ASSESS YOUR SITTING POSTURE

t work, are you a sloucher? Or do you perch on the edge of your chair? Do you sit on your foot or cross your legs? If even one of these is your habitual pattern, it can lead to distortions in muscle balance and to pain. Here is a way to rebalance.

How to do it:

1. Uncross your legs and place your feet on the floor or on your footrest.
2. Grasp your right butt cheek with your right hand and your left butt cheek with your left hand. (Yes, I did just say that.)
3. Lean over to your left side and gently pull the flesh of your right butt cheek to the right and slightly back. Sit back onto your right butt cheek. Then, lean over to your right side and gently pull the flesh of your left butt cheek to the left and slightly back. Sit back onto your left butt cheek.
4. It will have felt as if you spread your butt cheeks. (Yes, I just said that, too.)

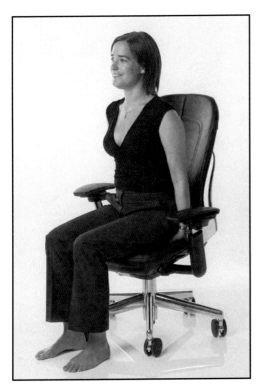

Flow fact:

In this position, your pelvis

becomes more neutral,

not rounded back or forward

or tilted too much to one side.

By doing this, the muscles that

connect from your pelvis to

your spine will be able to

come back into balance.

A number of students say that

this position alone has helped

reduce their back pain.

BEING ON THE BALL

xercise balls are becoming a popular addition to workplace furniture as a way of combining comfortable, pain-free sitting with a little bit of bounce.

1. ***Ensure a proper fit.*** Make sure the ball you are using is the right fit for you. When sitting on a properly sized, fully inflated ball, your knees and hips will be bent at about 90 degrees.

2. ***Fully inflate the ball.*** If the ball is not fully inflated, your knees end up being higher than your hips. This could lead to back injuries.

3. ***Maintain the natural curve of your spine.*** Feel your butt planted on the ball. Your sitting bones will feel equally balanced left to right, your feet flat on the floor, your head lifting toward the ceiling. If you are putting a lot of weight through your forearms onto your desk or wrist support, you are leaning too far forward. Reset yourself.

4. ***When you feel yourself slump, switch.*** Your body slumping signals fatigued muscles. This is your cue to move back to your conventional chair. When you feel refreshed, return to the ball.

5. ***Less is more.*** Remember, this is a workout. Sitting on a ball requires more from your muscles. Students even tell me they feel sore the next day. You may feel more action in your quadriceps, calves, abdominal area, or back. So, whether you are just starting out on the ball or you are a complete convert, stay aware of how your body is feeling.

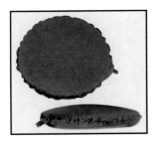

Not enough room in your workstation for both a ball and a chair? Try a tool such as the Active Disc. With properties similar to a ball, it is flatish like a pancake and sits directly on a chair. You will get all the benefits of being on a ball while sitting on your chair. Check out the resources section for suppliers.

Flow fact:

A sitting posture that

encourages natural

spinal movement

brings

clarity of thought.

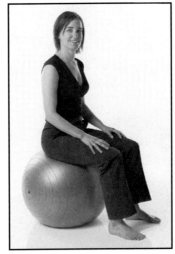

Practices for those times when
you think you have it all together
in the inner peace game,
and then . . .

Everything goes wrong ... then ... goes wrong again
What to do?
First . . . laugh, sigh, . . . scream . . .
at least you will know you are breathing.
And remember this quotation.

Peace.
It does not mean to be in a place
where there is no noise, trouble, or hard work. It means
to be in the midst of those things and still be calm in your heart.
– Unknown

Then . . . move your body . . . .

TWISTING TO REDUCE TENSION

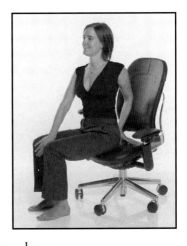

You've just gotten off the telephone with an irate customer, and now you're tense. Your neck aches and your back is getting stiff. What do you do to relieve the pressure? Twisting helps release tension that builds up along your spine. It also activates some of the muscles that contribute to developing solid core stability.

How to do it:

1. Sit facing forward, with both feet flat on the floor. Place your right hand on the inside of your right thigh, close to your knee.
2. Press your right hand into your leg so that your right arm is strong and your right shoulder blade gently moves down your back. Don't force.
3. Inhale softly. Exhale and gently twist to your left. Be sure your right shoulder is not popping forward by imagining that your chest is broad, with your collar bones wide.
4. This pose should feel light. As you exhale, come out of the twist. Repeat on the other side.

RELEASING YOUR JAW

ou've just had an argument with a colleague. Perhaps all that needed to be said couldn't be said (or wasn't said), and you are now feeling the tension sitting in your jaw or your neck, maybe in your eyes and forehead. Here is a way to release it.

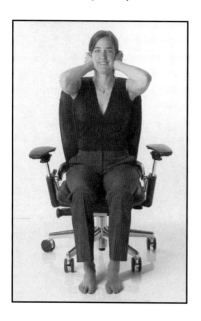

How to do it:

1. Move your fingers to your jaw joint (also known as the TMJ). To know that you are there, open and close your mouth. You will feel the joint moving under your fingers. Place the heels of your hands where your fingers were. Pressing firmly, but not hard, slide the heels of your hands along your jaw toward your chin.
2. Repeat if desired. You can also hold your hands statically in one position if it gives you a great release.

RIDING THE WAVE OF BREATH

The way you breathe can affect whether you become more or less anxious during stressful times. Typically, when stressed, the muscles of the chest and neck become tight, causing the breath to become held, or shallow. This limits the oxygen flow through the body and brain, causing more tension and possibly headaches, which in turn cause more stress. Here is a way to reverse that cycle.

How to do it:

As you breathe in, imagine the front of your body – chest, belly, and pelvis – relaxing, softening. Allow the exhale to emerge naturally. Continue the cycle for about 2 to 5 minutes. The result will have you feeling more centered, more at ease, and rejuvenated.

Flow fact: Research shows that using breathing techniques to help take care of your emotional health and well-being can make your physiological and biological age up to 16 years younger than your chronological age (from realage.com).

REDUCING EYE STRAIN

I t feels as if a heavy day has just sat on you, and you can feel the strain building in your eyes. You can tell it is going to create burning and tiredness in about half an hour. Here is a way to help prevent it from coming on full steam.

How to do it:

Eye strain is common at the end of a working day. The following exercises are best done as prevention before you feel the strain. Combine them with shoulder rolls (page 11) to ease neck and shoulder pain and to reduce the tendency for headaches.

1. Eyes closed – Up Down, Side to Side. *Be sure to keep your head still!*

    a) Raise your eyes to the ceiling, then drop them to the floor. Repeat four times.
    b) Move your eyes side to side. Repeat four times.

2. Eyes closed – The Clock. *Don't forget to breathe!*

    a) Move your eyes clockwise, then counterclockwise.
    b) Be sure to look at every "number" as you move your eyes around the circle.
    c) Blink your eyes gently four times when you are finished.

LEGS UP THE WALL

This is one of the most rejuvenating positions for desk jockeys. It can quell the anxious feelings that can spin around the heart, recuperate tired feet, ease lower back pain, and cultivate relaxation. It is also great to do if you wake up and your level of anxiety is peaking before your feet even touch the floor.

How to do it:

Find a wall space about the width of a door. Lie on your side, knees bent, with your butt about 6 inches from the wall. Roll onto your back, and let your legs move up the wall. You can stay in this position for between 1 minute and 15 minutes. Be sure to ensure the following:

- If, when your legs are up the wall, your butt is off the floor – even slightly – scoot back a bit so your butt comes back to the floor. This will help your pelvis be more stable.
- If the release feels too much like strain, scoot back. If you are not sure if it is a strain, notice your breathing. If your breathing is limited, scoot back.
- If your feet become tingly or numb-like, bend your knees and bring them to your belly. When the tingling or numb-like sensations go away, bring your legs back up the wall.

OBSTACLES AND HOW TO OVERCOME THEM

aving worked with "desk jockeys" for more than 7 years, I have heard many different obstacles, or reasons why people have difficulty doing the moves. The following is a list of common obstacles, as well as solutions for overcoming them.

1. I just don't have the time. This may sound familiar – "I have no time when I want to do yoga, and I have no desire when I have the time." There is a way to overcome this.

How to do it:

1. **Start small.** Begin with a time allotment you can truly commit to. Maybe it is 2 minutes over a lunch hour; maybe it is 5 minutes at the end of the day. Choose one or two of the practices on the preceding pages, ones that truly resonate or work for you, and practice those. If you practice, it will open up for you. That I can promise. But . . . you have to practice.
2. **Integrate the exercises into your day.** Try something similar to what Christopher does:

In your class, we were asked to take five deep breaths between each position. For some reason I have had trouble remembering to do this in practice at home. In order to make it a natural habit, I began taking five breaths between every task at hand during the day, and the consistency of the practice has served up a pleasant surprise. The breaths taken include the visualization that I am breathing through every pore in the body and the air is filling every cubic inch of this little old soul. Each time lately, whether in a meeting, a studio, or on the set, the five deep breaths are providing a cleansing, a relaxation, a centering, and a refocus of energy toward the next task or even the current situation. The beauty of it is that it can be done anywhere undetected, and in those situations where I can add a stretch or two, the benefit is immense. The benefits did not come right away, but after much "practice." So it would seem it requires a consistent repeated effort before those benefits appear. It seems to work a little better each day and has now become a habit of favour for me, or perhaps a coping tool for those tough days that everyone has.
– Christopher "Hap" Freeman

Or as Merri does:

The consistent thing I have been doing, since the seminar at our office, is the exercise where you envision that you are sitting on your hands [an adaptation of the exercise on pages 36–37]. I do this while on the C-train and sometimes (when I can think of it) at my desk. It has really diminished my lower back pain and also, as a little bonus, I feel it has helped my tummy muscles. – Merri Zickefoose

2. When I begin to practice, I all of a sudden remember all the things I have forgotten to do. So I stop to do them, then I never get to my practice. Here is a trick I used when I first started my meditation practice.

When I initially began my meditation practice, things at work and at home and other miscellaneous tasks would surface in my memory. Rattled by these thoughts, I figured it was more important to get these tasks out of the way, and that would calm my mind. So I would stop my practice to do them. The thing is I had created a habit – I kept stopping my practice. To change the habit, I started to keep a little notepad and pen by my side, so if something came up, I could write it down, and once it was down, I could refine my concentration on the meditation at hand. As my practice developed, there was less of a tendency to do this.

3. My mind chatter won't stop chattering. Remember that your mind is wired up to swing from thought to thought to thought. It is like a monkey that swings from branch to branch to branch, in a random, varied pattern. So as a novice to this practice, it may feel as if you are being invaded by your thoughts. Stick with the practice – notice the thought, then promptly come back to your breath. Chances are within the next three breaths, you will wander off again into the mind chatter. Again, just notice and bring yourself back to your breath. As you do this, it will become clear that the thoughts are just thoughts – thoughts of the past or future that have nothing to do with the present, this moment, now. Your breath, that is what is present. In time, you will begin to distinguish between what is present and what is mind chatter and more easily come back to the present.

4. I get tired or anxious when I do these exercises. When we begin relaxation or "getting present" practices such as these, the feelings or emotions we tend to suppress begin to bubble up. Why? Tiredness and anxiety don't often serve us during a working day – they get in the way of doing what needs to be done. As a result, there is a tendency to suppress them. Then, when you become quieter, through exercises such as those described in this book, the feelings and emotions that you suppress will start to come to the surface. (It is similar to those times when you are really busy and need to work "flat out," and then you go on holiday and get sick. You could feel yourself burning the candle to its bottom, but you had to suppress the feelings of tiredness and overwork in order to get done what you needed to get done.) What to do with them? Since they are giving you cues about your well-being, consider dealing with them however you need to – perhaps you need to rest, perhaps you need to visit with your doctor, or perhaps some other course of action is necessary. You'll know what you need to do. Just be sure you do it. *Soon.*

5. My work conditions are unsupportive of my practice. If your workplace culture doesn't support your taking a moment to move your body while at your desk, try what countless other desk jockeys have done – take your yoga to the bathroom stall.

6. I can't remember what to do. Keep this little book handy by your side, and you'll remember what to do.

7. I can't remember when to do it. Depending on the type of person you are, you may like to attach sticky notes to your computer; you may like to program your screen saver to say "breathe," "relax," "move your body"; or you may like to make a note of it in your Outlook or other time management system. You can visit our website to download e-cards and desktop wallpaper to help you remember.

8. *It is taking too long, and I don't feel I am getting it.* Here is a quotation from a director at Cirque de Soleil:

You can't hurry a learning curve. . . . You have to repeat and repeat and repeat a movement until it sinks into both your mind and your body. That's how dancers and acrobats learn.

– *Allison Crawford*

And so can you!!

Have a great day at work!

Susi

WOULD YOU LIKE MORE?

HERE ARE SOME RESOURCES TO HELP YOU BE PAIN FREE AND LESS STRESSED WHILE AT WORK

Ergonomic Resources

Balls or Active Discs can be a fun and safe alternative to sitting in a conventional chair. They are available at many retail stores. Fitter International produces a variety of sizes that are highly durable and burst proof; most have a lifetime warrantee. In Calgary, these products are sold out of their southeast location. To purchase online, visit **www.fitter1.com**.

For ***ergonomic consultations***, visit **www.iea.cc** for a listing of ergonomic consultants worldwide. In Calgary, connect with Shona Anderson at **www.anderson-ergo.ca**.

For ***ergonomic chairs and other functional office furniture and supplies***, visit RGO at **www.rgo.ab.ca**.

Yoga for the Desk Jockey™ Resources

Yoga for the Desk Jockey™ teaches yoga, breathing, and meditation techniques to people who want to relax, breathe, and move their bodies at work.

Yoga for the Desk Jockey™ – Online monthly ezine to your email account. This is a free ezine to help you continue to relax, breathe, and move your body while at work. Each month I send a technique specifically designed for you at work.

To receive the free Yoga for the Desk Jockey™ ezine, please visit our website at www.yogaforthedeskjockey.com.

Yoga for the Desk Jockey™ Lunch and Learns, Keynotes, Business Retreats

Thousands of participants have learned techniques from Susi Hately Aldous to help reduce the pain and strain from working at a computer, to feel more at ease and less stressed while at work. Her enthusiasm is contagious, making principles of yoga and stress reduction fun to learn and simple to apply to daily life. Her experiential workshops range from 1-hour sessions, to weekend retreats, to eight weekly sessions.

Here is a portion of what you will learn:

- A step-by-step process to relieve shoulder and neck pain
- A step-by-step process to reduce the effects of back and hip pain
- How to offset carpal tunnel syndrome
- Three key factors to ensure your workstation is set up properly for your body
- Breathing techniques to ease stress and strain and become more present
- How to access your intuition more clearly and easily

Yoga for the Desk Jockey™ Customized Yoga Programs
These programs are specifically designed for desk jockeys with pain, injury, or illness who want to cultivate relaxation, strength, and ease from the inside out. They are ideal if you feel your level of stress or busy work schedule is contributing to your health situation and you are looking for a way to transition yourself into a more balanced lifestyle.

Yoga for the Desk Jockey™: For your free time. In addition to helping you be pain free while in front of your computer, Yoga for the Desk Jockey™ offers additional support for when you are off of work.

For further details, please visit us online at www.yogaforthedeskjockey.com.

Spread the Word

Help a colleague release tension in their shoulders, back, neck, elbows and wrists. Order books for your employees, associates, suppliers, and clients. Easy to read, with plenty of practical applications. Special editions can be created specific to your organization.

For volume purchases sent to one address, **Yoga for the Desk Jockey** is offered at significant discounts with free shipping.

Please call or email us for details:

In Calgary: **403.229.2617**
Toll Free: **866.229.2645**
Email: **lovelyladies@ functionalsynergy.com**

TITLE	QUANTITY	PRICE	TOTAL
Yoga for the Desk Jockey		Price varies according to quantity	
Shipping and Handling			Varies depending on location
7% GST [Canada only: subtotal x 0.07]			
Total Enclosed			
GST registration number: 86446RT0001 Prices subject to change			

To order call 403.229.2617; Toll Free 866.229.2645

Check one: ☐ Visa ☐ MasterCard

Account #_____ Expiry Date _____

Cardholder's Name_____

Cardholder's Signature _____

  Or: Make MONEY ORDER or CHEQUE payable to:

      Functional Synergy inc

  Send to: #102, 6323 Bowness Road NW, Calgary, AB Canada T3B 0E4

DELIVER TO: Please print clearly

Name _____

Address_____

City _____

Province/State _____

Postal/Zip Code _____

Email Address _____

Telephone Number _____

About the Author

Susi Hately Aldous is an ergonomics consultant turned
certified yoga instructor. She combined the principles of yoga and
ergonomics to create the Yoga for the Desk Jockey™ workshop
and the globally read Yoga for the Desk Jockey™ ezine.
Her diverse background, which includes a BSc Kinesiology,
yoga certification, and practical experience in physical rehabilitation,
provides a functional and commonsense approach to her teaching.
Clients and participants say that Susi's style is
engaging, empowering, and loads of fun.
Susi lives in Calgary, Alberta where she owns Functional Synergy,
a yoga therapy website and consulting service designed to help people
overcome pain and injury so they can live the life
they want to live at home, work and play.